A Mother's Vaccine Dilemma

How to make your choice with confidence

Also by Trevor Gunn:

'Vaccines – This Book Could Remove Your Fear of Childhood Illness'
ISBN: 978-0-9928522-2-1
www.vaccine-side-effects.com

Trevor Gunn BSc Hons LCH ACHom
Medical Biochemist Registered and Practising Homeopath
www.achomeopaths.org

Currently At:
The Dyke Road Natural Health Clinic, Brighton, UK
www.dykeroadclinic.co.uk
And
The Japan Royal Academy of Homeopathy, London, UK
www.rah-uk.com

Trevor Gunn BSc Hons LCH ACHom
Can be available for talks & presentations
Please contact:
enquiries@trevorgunn.com
Trevor has presented in the UK, Ireland, Japan, Egypt, Lebanon, Iceland, Croatia and on National TV and Radio

A Mother's Vaccine Dilemma

How to make your choice with confidence

Trevor Gunn BSC Hons LCH ACHom

Published by

olistic
romotions

Holistic Promotions

ISBN: 978-0-9928522-1-4

Published & Designed by:

Holistic Promotions
202 Carterhatch Road
Enfield
Middlesex
EN3 5LZ
United Kingdom
email@holisticpromotions.co.uk
www.holisticpromotions.co.uk

Distributor:

Lightning Source UK Ltd
Chapter House, Pitfield
Kiln Farm
Milton Keynes
MK 3LW
United Kingdom
Fax: 0845 121 4594
www.lightningsource.com

CONTENTS

Contents

INTRODUCTION

For those parents aware that there is an alternative to simply 'saying yes' - the decision to vaccinate or not has become an immensely emotional and controversial one and in my experience it is a decision usually confronted by mothers. Although both parents will eventually contribute to the decision, most fathers have a natural tendency to go along with the prevailing medical advice, unless they are presented with overwhelming scientific evidence to the contrary.

But unfortunately much of the information vital to understanding the vaccine debate is in reality obscured from the general public, perhaps because of the acute sensitivity and emotion surrounding the topic. Consequently frontline healthcare professionals have a tendency to present the issues surrounding vaccination as being beyond question and unworthy of true scientific debate. Of course it's the mother who is usually in the forefront of this barrage of medical jargon and pro-vaccine statements.

It's against this backdrop that mothers who dare to question the safety or validity of vaccinating their babies can easily suffer from feelings of frustration, anxiety and isolation, at a time when the general challenges of motherhood are at their greatest.

Introduction

Many mothers have told me that the deep foreboding they have about vaccinating their child is nothing compared to having to survive the onslaught of orthodox medical opinion in response to any questions they may ask concerning the safety of our burgeoning vaccination schedules.

My name is Trevor Gunn I'm a graduate in medical biochemistry, a registered and practising homeopath. I have been studying this issue, treating children and adults for 25 years; I have also seen how vaccination issues have been blown out of proportion to keep many of the experts in control. However vaccines only relate to a tiny fraction of possible illnesses and so you may find that you're choices are actually simpler than you think. I am writing this book because I have learnt some valuable lessons about how to support children's immune systems and avoid chronic disease, and I would like to share this insight with you.

This book is a layman's guide to the main issues surrounding the vaccination debate, providing a foundation from which to ask insightful questions and make informed decisions. Basic principles are outlined so that the non-medically qualified can understand why the controversy exists, what alternatives are available and ultimately how to make your decision with confidence.

CHAPTER ONE

1   A Brief History of Germ Theory - The Rationale for Vaccines

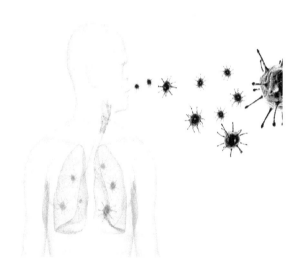

Chapter 1 Contents:

1.1 Pasteur and Béchamp

1.2 Why have we so heavily invested in germ theory?

1.3 Edward Jenner – The father of vaccination?

1.1 Pasteur and Béchamp

Initially we shall outline the rationale of vaccination by illustrating the kinds of diseases we vaccinate against, explain how our understanding of these illnesses have developed and show what options are available for prevention.

If we look back to the nineteenth century we can observe how much of our current medical ideas were developing - the time when scientific thinking began to dominate over many accepted religious beliefs, attempting to explain issues such as, how did life begin and how did we get here?

Two scientists in 19th century France, Louis Pasteur and Antoine Béchamp, were particularly interested in trying to understand disease processes, and two main schools of thought began to emerge. Pasteur held a 'creationist' view, believing that life and disease processes could happen from nothing – 'spontaneous generation'. Whereas Béchamp held a more 'evolutionist' view – meaning that disease processes evolved from what was already there.

Through his research, Béchamp discovered microscopically small organisms, what he termed 'microzymas' and that these were involved in disease (some of which we now know as micro-organisms). He discovered that these particles were already present within the healthy body and although sometimes associated with disease they need NOT have infected from outside of the body. In a suitable environment these micro-organisms could initiate fermentation, decay and disease by virtue of their living processes (metabolism). Even if they could be transferred from person to person they could ONLY reproduce in an appropriate environment.

Pasteur is often wrongly credited with having discovered that micro-organisms cause disease and that they can be transferred from person to person through the passage of air. The action of the microbe was however discovered by Béchamp and although micro-organisms; (bacteria, viruses, fungus etc.) can be transferred through the air, Béchamp made it very clear that the micro-organisms that are associated with illness are NOT the primary cause of the illness but merely accumulate if the conditions in the individual support those particular micro-organisms. In fact micro-organisms could live off a toxic internal milieu and can actually help to clean up the environment.

In approximately 1860 Pasteur, on seeing Béchamp's results, formulated the idea that for each particular process there must be a specific type of micro-organism responsible for the disease, this gave birth to his Germ Theory of Disease; again, a doctrine that had been formulated long before Pasteur had claimed it to be his own.

A fairly comprehensive summary of germ theory was postulated by M.A. Plenciz in 1762, <u>100 years before</u>

<u>Pasteur</u> had popularised it as having been his own, Plenciz stated:

> ***"There was a special organism by which each infectious disease was produced, that microbes were capable of reproduction outside of the body, and that they might be conveyed from place to place by air".***

According to 'germ theory' specific micro-organisms would cause specific diseases by entering the body from an external source, hence the term 'infection'; travelling from outside to inside.

These two interpretations of illness lead to very different views on the causes, treatment, and prevention of disease. If we are to accept Pasteur's theory, believing that the infecting germ is the most important part of the disease equation, then with regard to treating illness we would logically have to kill the germ or avoid contamination (i.e. avoid contact with anyone that has the germ), because it is assumed that the presence of the germ causes the disease.

Consequently the germ becomes synonymous with the disease; we talk about the germ and the disease as if they were the same thing.

Alternatively accepting Béchamp's theory requires that we understand that it is the individual's state of health, (their internal environment), that will affect the ability of the bacteria, fungus or virus to reproduce. The micro-organisms are already present and even if they could be transferred from one person to another the individual environment of each person determines the action of the micro-organism.

To improve health we must therefore improve the internal environment (the 'soil', the 'terrain', the 'milieu'). In addressing the human illness we need to look specifically at toxicity, diet and life-style, as well as ones mental and emotional state. If you change the 'soil', you will change the nature of the environment that the germs (micro-organisms i.e. bacteria, fungus, virus) live in, consequently you will change the type of germs present and you will also change the nature of the waste products that these germs generate, i.e. changing the soil will also change the toxins that the germs produce.

But it was of course the medical paradigm of Pasteur that we chose to adopt. There were certainly many social improvements made, but they came mainly as a result of social reform and rarely due to pressure from medical insight and since the nineteenth century our medical philosophy has stayed squarely within the doctrine of Pasteur.

1.2 Why have we so heavily invested in this Medical Paradigm?

There may be several reasons for this, one of which was not in fact the effectiveness of the approach;

there were many examples of communities and individuals adopting the Béchamp approach that were in fact more successful than Pasteur. However, it appears easier to blame a germ as being the cause of your condition and therefore easier to embrace the views of Pasteur, rather than acknowledging the real causes of disease, i.e. poor diet, toxins and life-style.

In the Pasteur paradigm, your illness was nothing to do with you and addressing your illness didn't require you to take any responsibility for your health or ill-health, psychologically it was easier to make Pasteur right and many wanted him to be right.

Also in the 19th century, the time of Pasteur and Béchamp was the time of the Industrial revolution and the social and economic conditions were appalling for the newly created working class. It was also standard medical text to acknowledge that the terrible living conditions were the causes of illnesses prevalent at that time. However, factory owners and land owners; the wealthy friends of government, were far too interested in profit to address the living and working conditions of the new working class. Economically and politically the medical paradigm of Pasteur received much greater support than that of Béchamp.

1.3 Edward Jenner – Father of Vaccination?

Turning briefly to Edward Jenner, he is commonly recognised as the father of vaccination. He apparently observed that once milkmaids had cowpox (a skin affection from the udders of cows), they would very rarely develop smallpox in later life. Jenner presumed that the immune response to cowpox was similar to the immune response to smallpox and therefore deduced that if you were immune to one you would be immune to both.

Edward Jenner therefore tried to create an extraction of cowpox, later termed a vaccination (vaccinia = Latin for cow) and inject this into individuals in the hope of stimulating an immune response to cowpox that would subsequently create immunity to smallpox.

Cowpox was seen as a milder disease than smallpox and it was hoped that vaccinating with cowpox would be a way of gaining immunity to the more 'dangerous' smallpox. In 1796 Jenner promoted this idea and the use of a vaccine, and the more popular history books credit Edward Jenner with the invention of vaccination. This procedure was however in existence throughout Europe at least 140 years before and in other parts of the world many years before that.

So in summary, according to Pasteur, we are assuming that diseases are caused by things (germs) that enter our bodies from the outside, and from the ideas of Jenner we are assuming that some of those germs are more dangerous than others. Each time we are handing more power to the germ, so that now the severity of the illness is also nothing to do with us but to do with the power of the specific germ.

However, a quick roll call of serious infectious illnesses may lead us to; polio, AIDS, meningitis, etc. and of the less severe; chicken pox, mumps, the common cold, even fungal illnesses. But a closer look will reveal that all of the so-called serious illnesses are associated with micro-organisms that many healthy people have within their bodies and they produce no symptoms at all - yes HIV, polio viruses, and the many micro-organisms associated with meningitis, (Hib, meningococcal, E.coli etc.) do not cause any symptoms in most people. In fact it is only in very few individuals that we even see symptoms.

With the so-called less severe illnesses... well, you can die from all of them, even fungal infections that can create mild symptoms in most, but can, and actually do kill others.

So although the medical paradigm with our 'germ consciousness' tells us that germs come and get us to cause disease and that some are dangerous and some are not; the reality is that any can be dangerous and all may not - clearly there is an issue of individual susceptibility that is totally missing from the germ theory of disease.

CHAPTER TWO

2 How Vaccines are Made and Tested

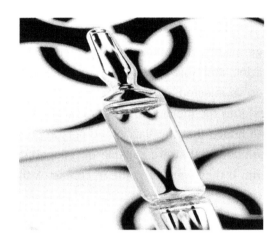

Chapter 2 Contents:

2.1   Vaccine Production in Principle

Edward Jenner tried to create a vaccine for smallpox from cowpox, using the pustule extraction of skin eruptions in cases of cowpox. However in modern-day vaccines we do not use a similar disease-causing germ to produce a vaccine but we use the actual germ that is thought to be responsible for a particular disease.

These germs are reproduced in the manufacture of the vaccine and this mixture of, germs and other additives, is injected (apart from the very few oral vaccines) into the individual in the form of a vaccine. It is then hoped that this vaccinated person produces blood antibodies that are capable of recognizing the real germ, if they were to come in contact with that germ later in life.

However in producing the vaccine, the pathogen (i.e. the germ or toxin that we place in the vaccine mixture) must be changed slightly, so as to avoid giving the person the actual illness.

This altered germ or toxin when injected into the individual will hopefully stimulate the person's immune system to produce antibodies, ones that are similar enough to recognise the real thing, and therefore work in a real disease situation.

However, if the pathogen is altered too much, in the production of the vaccine, then the antibodies produced by the administration of the vaccine will be too different to the original, and these antibodies would not recognise the 'real' disease pathogen. This is one of the inherent problems in creating vaccines; change the microbe too much and the immune response does not work against the real germ, don't change enough and the vaccine itself becomes very dangerous.

Vaccines can be live, killed, acellular and genetically engineered, but whatever the procedure the primary aim would be to stimulate the production of blood antibodies for a specific disease-causing agent (pathogen), which will hopefully remain in the body long enough to recognise and protect us from future contact with these pathogens.

2.2   Vaccine Safety

Most of the trials for the vaccines that are given to children are only conducted on healthy adults; this would therefore underestimate the impact of vaccines because children are more susceptible to toxins in vaccines than adults.

Secondly many of the initial vaccine safety trials were in fact only looking for symptoms of the specific vaccinated disease. For instance, if a measles vaccine was produced, whilst investigating the side-effects of the measles vaccine, researchers were only looking out for symptoms of measles. If a measles-kind of rash appeared in individuals it was presupposed that the vaccine would require further weakening and further investigation into the side-effects of this measles vaccine would be centred on looking-out for the symptoms associated with measles.

However, since then, we have discovered that vaccines can cause all kinds of symptoms, most of which were not being noted in these initial trials; therefore it is only more recently that we are realizing the serious consequences of vaccines.

Although vaccinators are using what they believe to be the cause of measles when they create the vaccine, the process of vaccinating, by injecting pathogens into the body is not the manner in which the disease is contracted naturally. It is actually more similar to a poisonous bite than natural measles; consequently the symptoms associated with the adverse effects of the vaccine are different than the natural disease you are vaccinating against.

The other problem with regards to safety is that there are strict time limits for the period in which reactions can be attributed to the vaccine. For example, with live vaccines you are allowed fourteen days to react, killed vaccines you only have 72 hours in which to react. If you react outside of these time periods then the adverse effects will not be acknowledged as being caused by the vaccine.

So this narrows the criteria in which we see adverse events, as many reactions may fall out of these time limits, some taking many weeks, months and years to fully manifest.

2.3   Vaccine Effectiveness

As for trials relating to the effectiveness of a vaccine, we need to be aware that the phase one trials that often publicise the effectiveness of vaccines tend to be test-tube studies, mainly concerning antibodies; these are often quoted as efficacy rates of the vaccine.

However these trials are inadequate, as they do not actually tell you what would happen in a real disease situation. Even if antibodies produced by the vaccine recipient do help in a real disease, there is a big assumption that they alone will protect the individual. The immune system is far more complex, and even now, still incompletely understood. For example it is possible to have high levels of antibody and not be immune. Equally it is possible to have no detectable levels of antibody and not get the disease. You may think that the medical profession would not agree with this.

The question with regards to antibodies and immunity was posed to Dr John Clements leader of the WHO EPI (World Health Organisation, Expanded Program on Immunisation) in a letter from me in September 1995.

Dr Clements agrees and it is recognised that an individual may have no or no measurable levels of antibodies and yet be immune to an illness. Similarly an individual may have high levels of antibodies and not be immune. Even back in 1950, a study of diphtheria conducted by the Medical Research Council in two areas of Gt. Britain found that despite having high levels of circulating antibodies some individuals contracted diphtheria, whilst others with very low levels did not.

In other words the presence or absence of antibodies in an individual is not an indication of immunity. It is not possible to test any one individual to see if they are immune or not by simply measuring their antibody levels. Antibody levels do not indicate immunity, and they are only a small part of your blood immune response, in fact with HIV, the presence of HIV antibodies is seen as the immune system's last resort, an indication of bad prognosis and a high risk of developing symptoms of AIDS.

UK health authority spokespeople often quote the measles vaccine as being 90% effective, this actually means that 90% of the recipients will produce the so-called 'necessary' antibody levels, 90% is not a measure of vaccine effectiveness in a real disease situation, therefore it is not a statement of how effective the vaccine is at preventing disease.

Similarly the necessary level of antibody as it relates to human illness is arbitrary, since there is no definition of immunity that can be defined from a certain level of antibodies.

This is especially important when considering that tests for immunity to rubella for example, which involves testing for blood antibodies and is often carried out to determine whether the individual needs the rubella vaccine or not.

However, the presence of antibodies to rubella virus would be indicative of you being exposed to the virus but that does not say whether you are immune or not, or if you became susceptible again that you would not get rubella. Similarly having no detectable levels of antibodies to rubella does not mean you are not immune. This is an important point to remember, especially if discussing this issue with your GP or health visitor.

CHAPTER THREE

3 The Evidence For Vaccine Effectiveness

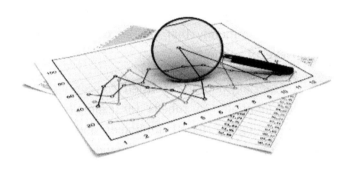

Chapter 3 Contents:

3.1 **Measles - Before and After Vaccines**

So if we can't tell from antibodies, how do we know that vaccines have worked? We are told that vaccines have eradicated disease, or have reduced the incidence of disease or reduced the severity of disease. That smallpox vaccine wiped out smallpox, and that polio is soon to be eliminated world-wide. The Department of Health book 'Immunisation against Infectious Disease' (1990/96 editions) illustrates the effectiveness of vaccines by showing the decline in incidence of disease after the introduction of the vaccines. For example:

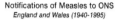

Notifications of Measles to ONS
England and Wales (1940-1995)

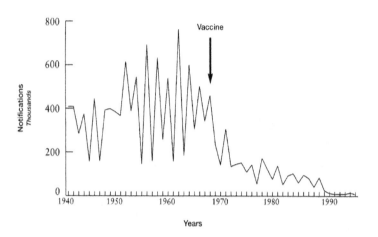

However to draw any worthwhile conclusions we need to see a 'before' and 'after', what was happening before the introduction of the vaccine?

However, as many of these illnesses were not notifiable diseases before 1950 (doctors were not obliged to report the numbers of people with these illnesses to their health authority) the health authorities are correct to say that they do not have reliable incidence figures before 1950.

So it's interesting to wonder how these figures are appearing in more recent publications.

However, we shall therefore look at the severity of illness as determined by mortality rates, that is, the numbers of people dying of a particular illness, which is an accepted indication of the severity of that illness.

Although this is a separate statistic from the incidence, in reality the incidence and severity statistics follow parallel and therefore similar trends. The following graph shows the rate of decline in mortality **before** the introduction of the measles vaccine.

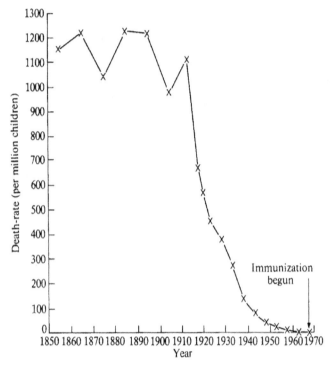

FIGURE 8.14. Measles: death rates of children under 15: England and Wales.

Looking at diphtheria, whooping cough, tetanus and tuberculosis, we can compare the graphs published by the UK health authorities showing data from 1950 with the OPCS graphs showing data from before that date, both are government offices.

3.2 **Diphtheria**

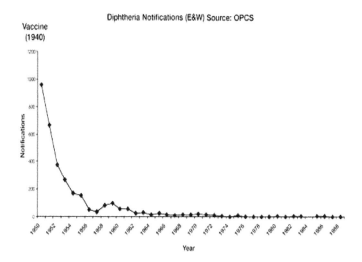

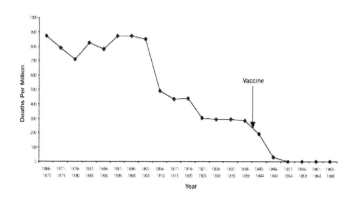

3.3   **Whooping Cough**

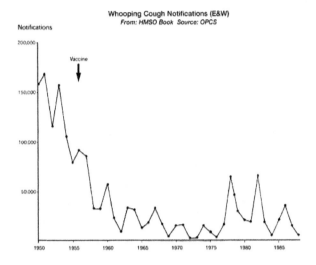

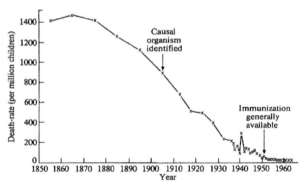

FIGURE 8.12. Whooping cough: death rates of children under 15: England and Wales.

3.4 **Tetanus**

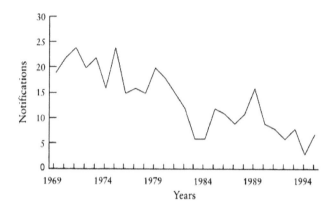

Tetanus notification to ONS
England and Wales (1969-1995)

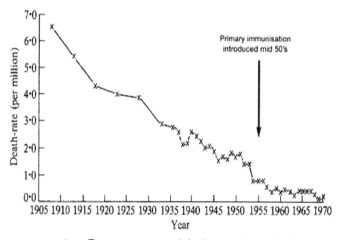

FIGURE 8.11. Tetanus: mean annual death rates: England and Wales.

3.5   Tuberculosis

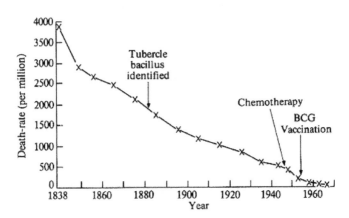

Notifications of tuberculosis and deaths to ONS
England and Wales (1940-1995)

———— Notifications

·········· Deaths

Respiratory tuberculosis: mean annual death-rates E&W.

These graphs all highlight the fact that the death rates for these infectious illnesses declined dramatically BEFORE vaccines were introduced. It is important to note that the statistics for these graphs are from the same government offices that collate the statistics for the graphs in the HMSO book promoting vaccines. They are not collated from studies carried out by people with different vested interests; the same departments that collate the stats for the HMSO book also have the statistics for the graphs shown here.

The main factors for these major declines were improvements in health brought about by improved nutrition, less over-crowded living conditions, clean water, sanitation, refrigeration of foods and so on. The healthier the population, the fewer cases, complications and deaths occurred.

3.6   Smallpox

In fact the only illness to have an increased death rate since the 1850's was in fact the first illness to be vaccinated against, smallpox.

In England: Free smallpox vaccines were introduced in 1840 and made compulsory in 1853. Between 1857 and 1859 there were 14,244 deaths from smallpox. After a population rise of 7%, the *death rate rose by 40.8%* to 20,059 between 1863 and 1865. In 1867 evaders of vaccination were prosecuted. Those left unvaccinated were very few. After a population rise of 9%, *the death rate rose by 123%* to 44,840, between 1870 and 1872.

The much touted anecdote 'vaccines have eradicated smallpox' cannot be justified by the actual evidence; in fact all of the evidence shows that the smallpox vaccine increased the severity and incidence of smallpox when all other illnesses (that at the time had no vaccines) were on the decline. Where do vaccine promoters get their evidence from, how much of this is just belief?

3.7   Scarlet Fever

The belief, that falls in vaccine uptake will result in huge outbreaks, does not make sense when confronted with the evidence. At the beginning of the 1900s scarlet fever accounted for the highest death rate amongst the childhood diseases, and yet this disease declined in the same manner as measles, whooping cough, tetanus, diphtheria and TB, such that now it is extremely rare. This achieved without the introduction of a vaccine; there has never been a vaccine for scarlet fever, it appears that the reduction in scarlet fever deaths and incidence just beat the pharmaceuticals to the post. Had there been a vaccine for scarlet fever, would we still be vaccinating against it now? Promoted by pharmaceuticals, exploiting the fear that it would ravage our children should we fail to vaccinate.

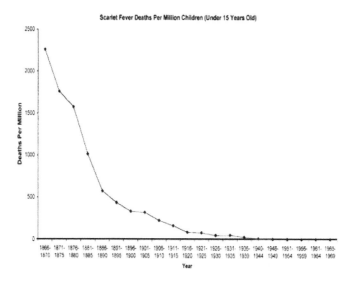

Scarlet Fever Deaths Per Million Children (Under 15 Years Old)

These graphs clearly show that factors other than vaccines affect health and therefore influence immunity to disease. Otherwise there would always be high levels of incidence and mortality, with falls occurring only when there was an introduction of a vaccine, and that is clearly not the case.

Often, vaccine promoters, talk of an unvaccinated child as an unprotected child, this is flawed science and a misrepresentation of the facts. You cannot 'unprotect' your child by not vaccinating, this presupposes that the only thing we have protecting us are vaccines, and as the graphs demonstrate, this is clearly not the case.

Natural immunity to disease is a natural consequence of general health promotion, you do not need specific vaccine-induced antibodies to be protected against disease, there are billions of microbes that are associated with illnesses that we do not have antibodies to and have not been vaccinated against and yet we do not develop illnesses to them either.

Factors that enhance natural Immunity have played the most significant role by far, in the reduction in severity and incidence of infectious disease. It is from this point that we assess the role of vaccines, how much more than natural immunity does a specific vaccine help me and is the potential benefit worth the risk?

CHAPTER FOUR

4 How Statistics Show Misleading Evidence for Vaccine Success

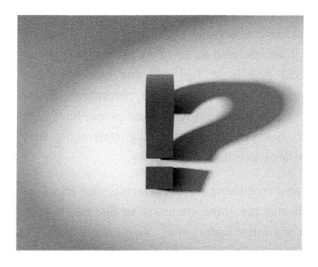

Chapter 4 Contents:

4.1 Epidemics

The word 'epidemic' conjures up quite an alarming picture in many people's minds ... 'An epidemic is coming', 'there's an epidemic just round the corner'. People tend to believe that if an epidemic hits an area or country then a high percentage will succumb to the disease. What is the actual definition of an epidemic?

An epidemic is actually quite small: for the case of polio it was defined as 35 cases per 100,000 people (0.035%) and is in fact less for other illnesses. Epidemics affect a very small percentage of the population which is not what most people have been led to believe through alarming statements from health departments and the media.

We know that there are many factors that affect our health and therefore immunity to disease, but are there any other factors that influence the statistics? What else can make it appear as though a particular vaccine is working, when in fact it may not be?

4.2 Reporting

The number of cases of disease recorded will not only depend on the actual number of people with those diseases, but just as importantly, will depend on the nature and accuracy of the reporting. There is a tendency to under-report the incidence of a disease in the vaccinated or in a community when vaccine uptake is thought to be high, and similarly over-report the disease in the unvaccinated or when the vaccine uptake is thought to be low.

For example, in the USA a television program, **DPT - Vaccine Roulette**, shown in April 1982, warned of the dangers of vaccination, especially the whooping cough component (the 'P' part of the DPT vaccine against diphtheria, whooping cough and tetanus) indicating it could cause neurological complications, brain damage and even death. Within months, whooping cough epidemics were reported in the states of Maryland and Wisconsin. It was stated by the Maryland Health Officials that the epidemic was due to parents seeing the documentary and not having their children vaccinated.

The cases were analysed by Dr Anthony Morris, an expert on bacterial and viral diseases and a member of the FDA (USA drug regulatory body). In Maryland, only 5 of the 41 cases were confirmed. In Wisconsin, only 16 of the 43 cases were confirmed.

Therefore whooping cough cases were being over-reported when the health authorities thought that vaccine uptake was low. However even more alarming was the fact that all of the confirmed cases had been vaccinated against whooping cough. A fact that had only come to light because of the investigation, Dr Morris therefore further concluded that whooping cough cases were probably occurring all the time in vaccinated individuals but were not being reported and therefore illnesses tend to be under-reported in the vaccinated. All of which would create a statistical difference in the numbers of illnesses in the vaccinated compared to the non-vaccinated due to a simple bias in reporting.

So the reliability of reporting in current society is highly questionable. Additionally, the immunisation status is often not highlighted or even established when we are told that vaccine uptake has been responsible for declines in disease or when reductions in uptake are blamed for the outbreaks of disease.

4.3   Disease Classification

The classification of a disease will have an impact on the number of cases of a disease. For example with polio, prior to 1955 if you had paralytic symptoms arising from a gut virus, lasting for over 24 hours, this would have been called paralytic poliomyelitis. However, after 1955 the paralysis had to last for anything from 14 to 60 days before it would be classed as paralytic polio. Since the majority of polio cases were resolved within a few days, then thousands of cases were reduced to dozens by this simple reclassification. An apparent fall in polio cases at a time that coincided with the introduction of the polio vaccine.

Also the system of classifying an illness according to the presence of a micro-organism brings certain problems and inherent inaccuracies. It is possible to have, for instance, a measles-like illness associated with viruses other than the measles virus, and paralytic polio-like illnesses associated with viruses other than polio viruses. We have now distinguished at least two viruses that are associated with symptoms of illness that are exactly the same symptoms as polio: the Coxsackie virus and Echovirus. They are part of a family of viruses of which we have now identified 72, all associated with symptoms that are exactly the same as paralytic poliomyelitis. Therefore, what would previously have been classified as polio will now be classified according to these new viruses.

There are also symptoms of polio that look like meningitis and if no bacteria are identified these cases would previously have been added to the numbers of cases of polio, whereas now all such cases are classified as aseptic meningitis. And where no microbe can be identified at all then the illness will be classified as Guillaine Barré syndrome.

So the effects of classification and re-classification of illness dramatically influence the numbers of cases of a disease giving an inaccurate epidemiology of the disease.

4.4   Symptom Suppression

Then last but not least the figures relating to the number of cases of an illness after vaccination do not tell you if the procedure of vaccinating has actually helped the population or created a deterioration in health.

For example, the mumps component of the MMR vaccine in the early 1990s was found to be causing mumps meningitis (and was eventually withdrawn). So it may have been possible to show reduced cases of mumps from a graph that only concerns itself with figures of mumps but if this was accompanied by increasing cases of meningitis then it is not possible to see this from such a graph.

This was only discovered after many years of vaccine use, so even if the vaccine could reduce the numbers of cases of mumps the important question remains, are we healthier or worse off as a result? Graphs showing declines in incidence of disease do not tell us what is happening to the whole health of the individual and therefore the whole population.

CHAPTER FIVE

5   Why Are Vaccines Not Tested Like Other Drugs?

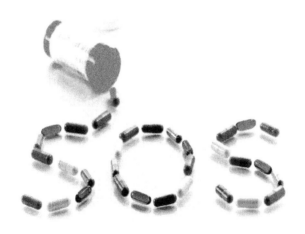

Chapter 5 Contents:

5.1   Vaccine Trials

To identify the benefits of vaccines as well as any associated problems, suitable trials must be conducted with long-term observations of vaccinated individuals. Designing such trials, would be relatively straightforward; we would need to have a control group, i.e. a group of individuals who are not vaccinated to compare with a vaccinated group.

There would need to be a large sample group and the selection of vaccinated and non-vaccinated would need to be made randomly, so that statistically you would be comparing groups with an equal variety of healthy, non-healthy, old, young, etc. The trial would also, have to be 'double-blind', meaning that neither the person administering the vaccine nor the recipient being vaccinated would know whether they were giving or receiving an injection containing the real vaccine or the non-vaccine.

It is important for both groups to think that they could be receiving the real vaccine or the non-vaccine. Because if people knew for example they were receiving the real vaccine and they had a positive association with being vaccinated, this would have an effect on the outcome. The belief in the benefit of the vaccine could positively influence your health and this is called the placebo effect. Almost all drugs that are used by the public have to go through some kind of double-blind, randomised, placebo, controlled trial.

5.2 Are Vaccines assessed like other Drugs?

Vaccines do not have to be trialled in this way before they are part of the public vaccine schedule since these trials are thought to be unethical. Why unethical? It is considered unethical to create a placebo group (an unvaccinated group) from which to make comparisons, as this would leave half of your sample group 'unprotected' and potentially exposed to a disease. But note, almost all other drugs are required to undergo this procedure.

Clearly the supposition is that the advantage of the vaccine must outweigh any disadvantage, and the vaccinated group would necessarily have an advantage over the placebo group. The pre-supposition is that the vaccine works better than placebo and the vaccines disadvantages do not outweigh any benefit. Then of course logically it would be unethical to create a non-vaccinated (placebo) group. But this is of course a circular argument, the point of the trial would be to determine that very premise; you cannot know that the vaccine benefits outweigh any disadvantage over and above natural immunity before you conduct a proper trial.

5.3 **Placebo controlled vaccine trial**

However one such study was reported in The Lancet, 12 January, 1980, the vaccine studied was the BCG vaccine against TB (tuberculosis). The trial involved 260,000 people comparing an equal sized vaccinated group with a placebo control group. This study was organized after various small studies conducted between 1935 and 1955, produced results that the Lancet states 'varied, strikingly and mysteriously, with protective effects ranging from 0% to 80%.' In fact those 20 years of trials were carried out after a vaccination campaign in a relatively small area of Europe left 72 children dead within a few months of inoculation with the BCG vaccine, a catastrophic event considering the low incidence of the disease and even lower death rate at the time.

The Lancet goes on to state that 'the largest controlled field trial ever carried out with this vaccine shows not only no evidence of a protective effect but in fact, slightly more tuberculosis cases have appeared in vaccinated than in equal-sized placebo control groups.' The results of the largest ever field trial carried out on BCG vaccine shows that you were more likely to develop TB had you been vaccinated, than had you not been vaccinated.

How did the authorities respond to such a result? We may have expected a re-trial at the very least, or further trials, perhaps a review of vaccine policy for TB and the withdrawal of the vaccine until, at the very least, the development of a better vaccine. However none of the above happened, vaccine policy continued regardless of the results of that trial.

Why was this? Would a proper assessment of vaccines be like opening Pandora's Box, a medical and political can of worms? Once you start, where would it end? Once you acknowledge ineffectiveness and side-effects, where would it stop, what would happen to the public perception of the pharmaceutical industry?

Medical professionals are like any other professionals, in that it is very difficult for them to question their core beliefs based on their training, practice and livelihood, even though the evidence suggests otherwise. But there are of course many that do question but find themselves constrained within a system that gives them very little alternatives to express and operate differently. Vaccines are viewed as one of THE medical wonders of modern medicine and it is often seen as medical heresy to even question them.

CHAPTER SIX

6 The Link between Toxins, the Immune System and Illness

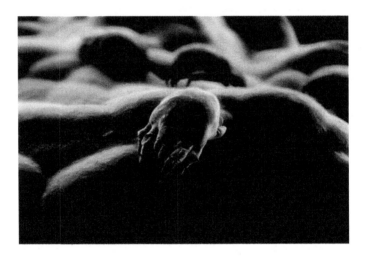

Chapter 6 Contents:

6.1 Immune Function & Toxicity

6.2 The Essential Role of the Skin and Mucous Membranes

6.3 Viral Illnesses

6.1 Immune Function & Toxicity

Let's now take a look at our physiology and the basic functioning of the body in a slightly more holistic manner than is common in our everyday medical language. In the diagram below we have illustrated a person with the mouth as shown; the mouth leads to a tube which goes into a bag, which is the stomach. The stomach leads into a longer tube, the small intestine. This eventually leads to the large intestine and finally continues out to your anus at the other

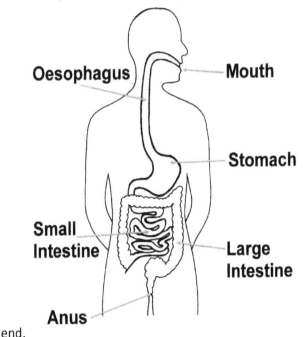

end.

In this simplified version of the body, we can imagine that whatever you put in your mouth is effectively still outside of your body, similarly what is in your stomach and intestines is effectively outside of the body. So for example, if you were to swallow a marble, at some time in the future after your daily evacuation, you would hear a 'chink' - and after the expulsion of that marble at no point did it go inside of your body.

It is only when something pierces your skin or the lining of your stomach and intestines (the skin around your body is continuous with the skin lining your stomach and intestines) that it enters the internal spaces of your body, with access to your blood, organs, nerves and so on. Now about 80% of your immune system actually functions in this 'outside space' of your body (stomach and intestines).

The Lungs

We could do a similar thing with your lungs; one tube leading to two tubes, ending in the convoluted membranes forming the membrane of the lungs. Gases pass in and out of the lung spaces, but it is only the substances that travel across the membrane that actually enter into your body.

The Bladder and Kidneys

Some toxins pass out of your body from your internal blood supply via the kidneys, across the membranes of the kidney tubules. One side of the tubule is your blood supply and the other side is the space that leads to your tubes that empty into the bladder. From here urine can then be expelled via the urethra - therefore once urine enters the space of the kidney tubules and bladder it is effectively outside of the body.

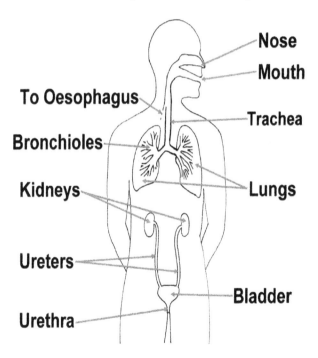

Toxins accumulated in the body are eliminated through the skin, the lungs, the kidneys and the large intestine.

Although we know these spaces are in intimate contact with the body and that substances can be absorbed into the body from here, the point is to create a perspective of how the body functions in eliminating out into these spaces and how important these actions are in immune function and in maintaining health.

6.2   Skin and Mucous Membranes

So the body has the permanent job of keeping things out that it does not want, and eliminating naturally produced waste (that it similarly doesn't want). This barrier keeping unwanted things out and eliminating toxins carries out a large part of our immune function and the main structure involved would be the skin or mucous membrane. Now there are many components associated with those membranes:

- White blood cells (immune cells) that can enter any part of that system. They have access to your lymphatic vessels and glands such as tonsils and adenoids

- Non-specific antibodies

• Bacteria that help your immune system to function (there are *more* micro-organisms in your body than there are your own cells)

• Hairs that filter

• Enzymes able to break down components

• Immune chemicals that coordinate and carry out immune function

• Mucus fluid that can be acidic or the opposite alkaline

• The membrane itself functions as the most important barrier

So when there is a toxic problem and/or an abundance of non-beneficial microbes, these elements operate at the site of toxicity breaking down and digesting unwanted material so that they can be eliminated from the system.

6.3   Viral illnesses

Since the discovery of microbes, such as bacteria, we have seen similar diseases that are not associated with bacteria. Consequently there are whole classes of illnesses that are thought to be caused by smaller microbes called viruses. However, contrary to the public portrayal of illnesses, the idea that viruses are actually the cause of illness by taking over and killing cells is still a very inadequate theory.

Standard immunology books will state that we are still uncertain as to how the immune system deals with viruses and most viruses we study live with their host cells without causing disease. There is more evidence to suggest that viruses are broken down elements of cells and therefore part of the clean-up process; because we know that viruses can be caused by poisoning cells with various toxins. So it is possible to create viruses within you, by poisoning your cells.

Also we have never been able to prove that viruses cause illness even with our modern technology able to detect viral particles. Such infecting viruses (infectosomes) have never been demonstrated in diseased tissue.

It's rather like flies around cow dung, in many instances they are there but they don't actually produce the cow dung.

CHAPTER SEVEN

7 A More Holistic View of Disease

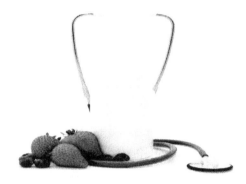

Chapter 7 Contents:

7.1 Distinguishing the Problem from the Reaction

A child's system, from birth, is of course immature and in the early stages of development.

The stomach and intestinal membranes are more porous (leaky) than the adult membranes, thereby allowing things into the blood far more readily than in an adult.

Therefore a baby will be initially fed baby milk, ideally breast milk, which has small nutritional components that do not need much breakdown and digesting, these elements are beneficial and will be absorbed very easily across the membrane and therefore into the body of the child.

What would happen if you gave your baby *'meat and two veg'* from birth?

This would poison the child, due to the inability of the child to digest the food; they do not have the necessary enzymes to break down these large food molecules, and their membranes are unable to keep out all of these elements from the blood, effectively resulting in toxins entering the blood.

So how would the child react to ingesting a potential poison? Initially babies react typically through vomiting and diarrhoea, they don't initially even have the capacity to create a fever, it may take days or even weeks for some babies to develop the capacity to have an inflammatory response.

The 'reaction', vomiting and diarrhoea, is therefore a necessary part of the resolution of the problem of toxicity in the gut. Therefore the 'problem' is the toxin accumulation in the digestive tract and the 'reaction' vomiting and diarrhoea, is part of the cure.

7.2 Suppressing Reactions Can Lead To Deeper Problems

However, often the current pharmaceutical orthodoxy perceives the vomiting and diarrhoea as being the problem itself, rather than being the reaction to the problem, so often the problem and reaction are treated as one. In fact generally the real problems are ignored and the reaction itself is seen as the dangerous thing to be stopped. Consequently medication is taken to suppress reactions in an attempt to treat the condition, i.e. drugs to stop diarrhoea and vomiting.

Logically, suppressing the very reaction needed to resolve the problem will make it more likely that the problem remains i.e. in the case of toxic build up in the digestive tract, those poisons will remain in the digestive tract, which will lead to either a recurrence of the reaction (vomiting and diarrhoea) or the body will step-up it's attempt to resolve the situation.

7.3 Inflammation, Stepping-up the Reaction

The next step would take the form of an inflammatory response, if the child is able to do this. An inflammatory response is the mechanism whereby the body mobilizes white blood cells to an area of toxicity or dead/injured tissue. To do this, the blood vessels widen in that area, (called dilation). Secondly the membranes separating the blood from the toxic space (in this instance the gut membrane) and the blood vessel walls themselves become more permeable (leaky), allowing the white blood cells to squeeze out of the blood vessels into the relevant space of the body, leading to symptoms of redness, swelling, pain and heat.

The white blood cells once in the appropriate place will break down/digest toxins and dead tissues, preparing them for elimination; again via the process of vomiting and/or diarrhoea. There is a general movement of immune cells out of the body into the gut space, remember the area of the gut is considered to be outside of the body.

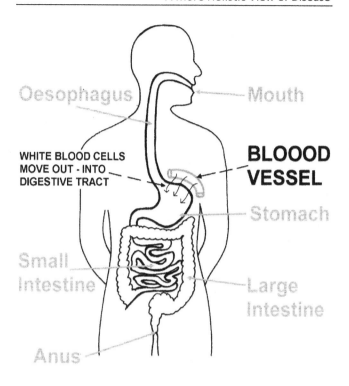

The aim of the body's response is to keep the toxins out of the bloodstream. So your child's body will mount an inflammatory response at the appropriate site, maybe as a gastritis, laryngitis, sinusitis, cystitis, and so on, to keep the toxins outside the body. Again it is possible from an orthodox medical perspective to perceive the inflammation as the problem itself, giving anti-inflammatories to suppress these reactions.

Consequently if toxins are not eliminated from these external spaces, (external from our previous definition including the respiratory, digestive, and urinary tracts) what then happens to them?

7.4 Crossing the Membrane Leading To Blood Elimination

In intimate contact with the membranes and without elimination, they have the potential to pass across the membrane and get into the blood, it is also likely that toxins that naturally accumulate in the blood as a result of our normal metabolism build-up within our internal blood system; this then leads to a very different reaction in an attempt to cleanse the body once again. Here we see the mobilization of other white blood cells, in the blood itself;

T-cells, B-cells, Natural Killer cells and in some instances the production of antibodies, produced by the B-cells.

You could have white blood cell reactions, which tends to deal with the cells that have been affected by the toxins. If these cells fail to deal with the problem, for example, if toxins remain in the blood, then antibody production is called for. Antibodies appear to be the last line of defence for your blood system, and may not be required if the body's cellular immune response is successful, and the required elimination takes place. Antibodies themselves do not destroy anything or eliminate anything, they act as flags indicating where potential problems remain, attracting other elements of the immune system to do their work.

Normally when the toxins are eliminated from the blood they will be eliminated through the skin and/or mucous membranes resulting in rashes. Diseases with skin rashes, such as measles, rubella and chickenpox, etc. are good examples of what orthodox medicine calls *'viral shedding'*.

The importance of this skin elimination of toxins has been demonstrated in an orthodox medical study carried out in Denmark and reported in The Lancet, 5 Jan. 1985. The initial research looked at a group of adults who had measles-specific antibodies present, this meant that they had been in contact with the measles virus but this was not a statement as to whether they were immune or not.

Comparing those cases which had produced a typical rash with those cases that did not, the evidence showed that the <u>absence</u> of rash increased the incidence of; skin diseases, degenerative diseases of bone and cartilage and certain tumours in adulthood. It was therefore deduced even from an orthodox perspective that the rash, the elimination process, the viral shedding, is an important part of the resolution of illness and should not be suppressed.

7.5   Immunity as a Learning Process

So far we have looked at immune responses as 'processes' and therefore it is important to realize that 'immunity' is not a 'thing', it is the result of a system going through a process. If the immune response is to be more able to cope with conditions after that process, with enhanced immunity, then the system has to 'learn'.

Thinking of the immune system as the possession of chemicals such as antibodies would be like saying education is about having books, but giving children lots of books does not make them educated. The process of learning to read must take place first. Immunity is not a set of things like a bunch of antibodies, things that you would like to give to an individual; it is a learning process that the body goes through, which results in the person becoming immune i.e. less susceptible to illness.

We are now able to understand that the immune system learns as do many other systems in the human body. This learning process educates and primes the body for future events. It is the same when your child is learning to walk. When ready to learn to walk the initial phase involves standing up, they do inevitably fall down. Much as we would like to teach our children without them falling, we inherently know that this is not possible; learning takes place by a process of trial and error.

We therefore minimize the consequences of error, (soft flooring, no dangerous items to fall on etc.), however, we cannot eliminate the possibility of error and therefore we reduce the consequences but not the risk of actual error. So after the fall, first the child learns to get up again, the consequences of error, the fall has not been so damaging that the child is unable to try again, so the error of falling is resolved and the child stands again. At some point however we expect the child to learn to balance and that is the point of learning. After learning the child is now less susceptible to falling. If the child had learnt to walk and fallen such that they were seriously injured and shocked, that would have made them less able to get up after and in fact more susceptible to falling.

Likewise when the body eliminates toxins, if there was no learning then the body would be just as susceptible to that toxic build up in the blood system as it was before, like a child that never learns to walk always standing and falling, the body would forever be having rashes and measles. However with real immune learning not only do immune cells learn but the most important elements of the immune system i.e. the membranes also learn. They learn to keep things out that it previously could not i.e. the integrity of the membrane gets stronger, it becomes less penetrable.

So you often find that once you have had certain illnesses you are much less likely to suffer from them again and additionally many aspects of the immune system will have been strengthened. This learning is what we call immunity, but it is not rigidly specific, as we initially believed when we thought that specific antibodies were necessary for immunity. However the non-specific nature of immunity is in fact just like any learning, once your child has learnt to walk in one room they can walk in another room, or learnt to cross the road they can cross another i.e. there is some specificity but also considerable overlap in our learning capacity.

If that was not the case then we would have to have every single illness possible to become immune to all of those illnesses, and that doesn't happen and is not necessary.

It is often asked, why did indigenous people succumb so readily to illnesses of their invaders, for example, with the South American Indians with the landing of the Europeans? Here we need to be aware of the distortion of events to suit a prevailing theory. When Europeans landed in South America there were many atrocities carried out to the local people, violence, killing, rape, destruction of homes, stealing resources, enslavement, lifestyle and dietary changes imposed, to name but a few. If we study disease we see they are caused by certain conditions, as would be expected in the above example.

In more recent times when there are visitors from developed countries to cultures that are subsequently newly exposed to our so-called viruses, we see there is no increased susceptibility to disease. If we really are visitors performing acts that are no more detrimental to our hosts than breathing on them and sharing air-borne microbes, then no disease is created.

7.6   Chronic Disease is a Persistent Response

It is important to realize also that unresolved issues lead us to become more susceptible to our problems. If we look at an emotional example, let's imagine a child on their first day away from their parents, at school. They experience the trauma of 'separation', and they may react by 'crying', if the expression of their grief, crying, was suppressed i.e. they were told not to cry, made to feel afraid to cry, then the very reaction that helps them to resolve the situation has been suppressed. The problem has of course not been resolved, in fact the problem stays within, and the child becomes sad.

Here we demonstrate that if the acute reaction is unsuccessful, it leads to a chronic reaction, the acute is intense and short-lived and the chronic is less intense and long-lived. Whilst in that state of sadness and unresolved grief, the child is in fact more susceptible to separation trauma. Even within their home, with their parents, they may even get upset when being left alone in a room as a result of this unresolved issue. Unresolved issues lead therefore to chronic weakness.

To continue our story of immune function, if the elimination of blood toxins is unsuccessful then we will observe the build-up of toxins in internal parts of the body, joints, fat, kidneys, liver, and heart valves. This may then lead to inflammatory conditions in those areas, but it may also lead to chronic reactions, vomiting and diarrhoea lead to chronic digestive disturbances; an acute rash could become a chronic rash, (eczema); an acute cough becomes a chronic respiratory illness (asthma).

If we look a little closer at our generalised inflammatory response to blood toxins, we see that during the inflammatory process it is important to get your white blood cells to the appropriate areas and eliminate blood toxicity out, beyond the mucous membranes and skin.

To accomplish this, the membrane becomes more permeable, (more leaky). However, this is part of the 'acute reaction' and when the situation is resolved we would expect the membranes to return to the original state and if there has been a positive learning, then the membranes do in fact become stronger as a result of the process.

CHAPTER EIGHT

8 What Really Happens To The Body When You Vaccinate?

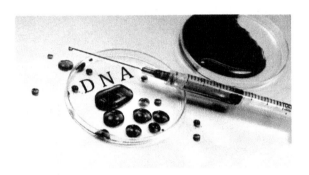

Chapter 8 Contents:

1. Vaccines Bypass Most of the Immune System

2. A Little Poison Helps the Medicine Go Down

3. Vaccines are always contaminated

4. Antibodies - A Partial Immune Response

5. Stimulate to Suppress

6. So what is the Significance of Leaky Membranes?

8.1 Vaccines Bypass Most of the Immune System

Vaccines introduce their antigens and other chemicals directly through the skin and therefore straight into the body with access to the blood, organs and nervous system. It is estimated that 80% of immune cell activity occurs on the membranes of the digestive tract, there will of course be more activity on the membranes of the skin, lungs and urinary tracts. The membrane itself performs a vital barrier and therefore immune function, so it is easy to recognise that a vaccine does in fact bypass most of the immune systems of the body. Therefore vaccines only stimulate a very small element of the immune system and do not replicate the immune learning that develops from naturally acquired immunity

8.2 A Little Poison Helps the Medicine Go Down

In looking at the vaccine process with relation to microbes that are thought to cause diseases, it is interesting to note, that if we were to inject somebody with just these killed or live microbes, one would expect the body to produce lots of antibodies to deal with this threat. But actually, very little happens; microbes injected into the body are not a natural phenomenon, it may be that the body simply doesn't recognise what is occurring, the microbes haven't entered in a way that would naturally happen in disease. Similarly some viruses themselves may not be the causes but results of disease, so once again the body does not see this as a significant threat, especially again if the virus has been changed in some way.

Therefore to actually get the body to respond to the vaccine, a poison is put in the vaccine specifically to kick the immune system into reacting, this poison is called an ***adjuvant***. Aluminium phosphate or aluminium hydroxide is usually used in the early baby vaccines for this purpose; to get the body to react. This has just as many potential problems associated with it as mercury, which for a long time was denied as causing problems, and was eventually reduced in some vaccines for the very reasons that were originally denied.

8.3   Vaccines are always contaminated

Another inherent problem with vaccine production is the cultivation of virus which for the vast majority of vaccines involves growing the virus on animal tissue. Polio virus, for example, is grown on monkey kidney cells and one of the problems with cultivating viruses is that, as the specific virus is replicated, other things will grow too. This creates the issue of contamination; it is actually not physically possible to produce a pure virus, therefore all viral vaccines have a level of contamination that is allowable. The amount of contaminant virus numbers into millions, and some of these artificial contaminants do create problems in humans that may not be apparent in the animal tissue that it has been cultivated on.

For example, the polio vaccine has been known to be contaminated with a cancer-causing monkey virus called SV40, since the 1950s, the contamination was allegedly rectified but debate as to liability still continues to this day.

Vaccine virus also needs to be weakened or killed using physical or chemical procedures; the vaccine also contains preservatives, antibiotics, stabilisers, and elements of the genes of the tissue that the virus was cultured on. This results in a cocktail of components that have the potential to cause a wide range of health problems.

8.4 Antibodies - A Partial Immune Response

By vaccinating you basically introduce a foreign cocktail of chemicals into your blood and leave them there. The idea is to produce antibodies, as the possession of antibodies was thought to be immunity, but this is an old (pre-1940) idea of immunity. But having blood antibodies no more constitutes immunity than the possession of books constitutes education. Anti-bodies flag up elements that you need to eliminate from the body, if the toxins are not eliminated the immune process is in fact unresolved and there is no immune learning.

8.5   Stimulate to Suppress

Worse still, if a person does produce an immune reaction to a vaccine, with for example a fever, i.e. an attempt to mobilize white blood cells with a generalized inflammatory response, then the fever is routinely suppressed with antipyretics and anti-inflammatories such as calpol, paracetamol etc.

This is in fact an illogical and dangerous procedure; on the one hand you want to stimulate an immune reaction by injecting poisons into the body and at the same time you are asked to suppress the immune reactions. If this does lead to unresolved immune responses we may expect to see an increase susceptibility to illness not a decrease as you would obtain with a legitimate immune learning. One of the ways of demonstrating this, from a physiological point of view, would be to study what happens to the membranes of the body after vaccination.

It has been demonstrated and reported in medical literature that vaccines can cause certain blood chemicals to persist long-term in the body; chemicals that should only be there in acute disease (i.e. short-term). (Henry Pabst in the case of MMR ['*Vaccine*'-15:1;10-14]). Therefore in response to vaccines we are seeing chronic long-term reactions, and in addition the membranes have been shown to be persistently leaky.

We are observing chronic disease reactions in response to vaccination because clearly the child's body finds it extremely difficult to eliminate poisons that have not entered the body in the manner that we have evolved to deal with, and secondly any attempt to actually resolve this is usually suppressed.

8.6   So what is the Significance of Leaky Membranes?

If you have persistently leaky membranes you become more susceptible to substances getting across your membranes and into your body, food substances, elements in the air we breathe and toxins gain access to your blood and internal systems. If you cannot eliminate these things and keep them out, you become sensitised to them. As such allergic reactions are in fact not over-reactions but damage limitation strategies designed to stop further intake of a substance that has already gained access to your blood system.

If we take an emotional example; a child exposed to an acute trauma, such as a strong act of violence. The child is unable to accommodate this in their psyche and they cannot deal with the levels of fear it creates, however the effects of the trauma will remain there until it can be resolved at a later date and in the meantime they become sensitive to any violence or anything that looks like violence. So if they saw somebody approaching that could appear to be menacing they may appear to be over reacting and that is what is meant by sensitised. It may appear like an over-reaction, but for that individual it is an appropriate strategy given the unresolved trauma within.

When a vaccine is introduced into the blood, the membranes can become more leaky and the system sensitised to the elements within the vaccine. Vaccines contain many elements; foreign proteins, antibiotics, metals, additives, contaminant viruses, foreign genes and preservatives, which have the potential to cause various sensitivity reactions in some individuals.

When a person develops an allergy, this allergy is the result of something that has been given access to the blood. If you are allergic to egg protein this means that egg protein has or is getting into your blood and you cannot get it out - you have become sensitised to egg protein. Usually you find that people with allergies are sensitive to many things, as it is rare to have an allergy to just one thing.

The body then produces another type of antibody and places it on the part of the body that will meet the substance first, i.e. the skin, mouth, nose etc., the body is then instructed to react strongly if there is any contact with that substance, so as not to allow intimate contact with lungs, digestive tract etc. The body knows that if that substance has access to the membranes it will get in and cause problems in the blood. For example, we think 'pollen is not dangerous', so hay fever must be an over-reaction; however pollen is dangerous in the blood, therefore more dangerous to people with an allergy to pollen.

Large protein molecules, especially from foods, are in fact dangerous in their whole unbroken state in the blood. If we then take antihistamine to stop that reaction then once again the antihistamine drug suppresses our highly evolved damage-limitation reaction, i.e. the allergic reaction, and we allow more of the problem into the blood to affect the internal systems of the body. Until eventually the allergic reaction itself does create a problem.

CHAPTER NINE

9 What Makes Us Susceptible to Illness?

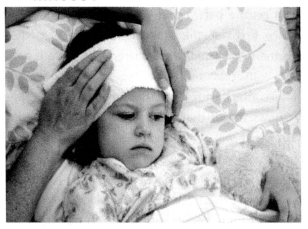

Chapter 9 Contents:

9.1   Susceptibility and Microbes

In order to understand how people become susceptible to contracting illnesses, including the so-called infectious illness, we need to look at certain issues from a more holistic point of view.

The human being 'reacts' to trauma or stresses in order to resolve their impact on the body and where possible to 'learn' from the process.

Therefore the symptoms are not the problems in themselves; they are often part of the solution. It is the traumas & stresses, that illicit the symptom-reactions that are in fact the problems. The traumas are often associated with life-style, diet, environmental toxins, mental and emotional stresses, etc.; often we need to address and reduce these in order to resolve illness.

We react in ways that are unique to us all and this is called our 'susceptibility'. Issues that are not resolved remain and influence our future reactions to stress, the patterns of these unresolved illness may also be passed on to future generations.

Microbes (bacteria, fungus and viruses) although involved in the manifestation of infectious illness often aid in the breakdown of diseased tissue and toxins, many are the *result* of disease not the primary *cause*. Microbes do not cause serious illness by virtue of the type of bacteria, fungus or virus. The type of illness is determined by ones individual susceptibility. Which is why most people have no symptoms even though we all harbour microbes that can be associated with serious infectious illnesses such as meningitis, encephalitis and septicaemia etc. They are only associated with serious illness if we are seriously ill. Serious illness comes from unresolved issues, which are ultimately caused by severe or persistent trauma and/or persistent symptom suppression.

Therefore as you raise your level of health you become susceptible to different, less severe types of illness, whether you are exposed to bacteria, viruses and fungus or not. There is no such thing as a dangerous microbe, just dangerously ill people.

This is a very different way of understanding disease for many people in orthodox medicine and consequently for most of the media and general public, but not so for most in holistic medicine. But you have only to stop and think about the reality of infectious agents such as bacteria and viruses etc. to realise that the issue of individual susceptibility is of ultimate importance.

All previous attempts to scare and all previous fears of illnesses have never materialized in the manner predicted by those that promote the idea that the disease is determined by the germ; Sars, Bird flu, HIV, Ebola, all illnesses for which we have no effective treatment or drugs to destroy the virus and yet these illnesses did not wipe out large sections of the community as predicted but merely stayed within a very small section of susceptible people. Having the *illness* and having the *microbe* are clearly two entirely different things.

From a pharmaceutical point of view we are taught to be afraid of all illness, that immunity can only be obtained by having the illness, that some illnesses are too dangerous to come in contact with and if we are exposed to a new germ (from an illness we have never had) we are likely to contract the illness.

Consequently we are being vaccinated for an ever-growing number of diseases, and by the very nature of this theory the number of vaccines recommended will inevitably continue to increase. There has been a 700% increase in vaccines given to children in the UK over the last 50 years, a trend that is mirrored around the world.

The medical profession as directed by the pharmaceutical industry presupposes that we require specific antibodies to every microbe in order to be protected from their associated illness, and as discussed earlier, antibodies only play a small role in immunity and their mere presence does not mean that you are protected.

9.2   Consequences of acute illness

There are certain consequences to having acute diseases, (an acute illness being a reaction to an imposed trauma/stress), two of which we have already discussed:

- Resolution - leading to learning
- Unresolved - leading to chronic disease.

However we can in fact distinguish four main outcomes of acute disease as follows:

1. The trauma is resolved and you have learnt from the process, your health improves to a higher level than before, therefore *less susceptible* to the trauma.

2. You resolve the acute but carry on as before, just *as susceptible.*

3. The problem is not resolved and your health deteriorates to a lower level than before and you are therefore *more susceptible* (sensitised).

4. The problem is not resolved resulting in death.

From observing patterns of illness, holistic therapists have also observed that these unresolved patterns can be acquired in one generation but can also be passed on to the next generation. Therefore according to the nature of the parent's development through their life-time, their later children may be healthier or less healthy than their older siblings.

We find that the children who express their acute illness become healthier and less susceptible to other illnesses, allergies, asthma, and so on. Whereas those who have their acute disease suppressed are more likely to deteriorate and become more susceptible to other conditions. This is an observation of symptom patterns from over two hundred years of cases from many thousands of practitioners and is in line with later research studying those issues:

> On June 29, 1996 the Lancet reported on medical studies showing that children with a history of natural illnesses such as measles, mumps and rubella were less likely to suffer with **allergies** in later life. Researchers from Southampton General Hospital in the UK now confirm this, discovering that: Children with a history of measles suffer less from allergic conditions such as asthma, eczema and hay fever when compared to vaccinated individuals.

Holistic therapists are trained to make observations and notes of all symptoms, in order to understand a child's health. Holistic therapists also look at the parents' and grandparents' health, which is why your practitioner will ask about the family medical history. This enables the practitioner to understand the child's level of health and potential patterns of illness that may have been inherited. We may inherit more from one parent than the other but can only start with a level of health as great as the healthiest of one of our parents.

As each generation's health declines the inheritance will also change. Nowadays you will find more children developing cancers at a very early age, whereas in previous generations it would take longer to develop such chronic disease. Many children of today are starting at lower levels of health due to the unresolved issues of the parents.

The expression of illness, the elimination of toxins and immune learning are the goals of the holistic practitioner. The aim is to get the body functioning to allow the elimination of stored toxins and to allow the resolution of stored trauma.

9.3 Susceptibility to Infectious Illness

Regarding the resolution of so-called infectious disease, a holistic practitioner will be looking for toxin elimination. Generally there are three components to what we are told is an infection:

> 1. The development of the immune system i.e. the ability of the body to eliminate and to get stronger.

> 2. The amount and the location of toxicity in the system.

> 3. The amount of existing chronic disease, i.e. the unresolved issues carried by the individual.

An acute infectious illness is a crisis of toxicity, that may come about under times of stress; emotional and/or physical. If resolved it may enable immune learning and may also help to resolve unresolved patterns that have been inherited and/or acquired. As a consequence of these potential issues, illnesses will therefore express differently in different individuals.

The same potential illness, associated with the same pathogen will be expressed differently in different individuals because we all have varying degrees of health and chronic disease. Polio virus is associated with a whole host of symptoms from virtually none, to minor digestive complaints, to spasm, to paralysis, to brain disorder, to death; the virus is exactly the same in all cases; the difference is due to the differences in susceptibility of the patient.

If the elimination process is suppressed then toxins can move *deeper within the body* causing more serious consequences. This can result in a reduced ability to eliminate and at this point your body is less able to resolve that illness with an acute disease reaction and may ultimately lead to a chronic disease. Some people are in fact not healthy enough to have symptoms of measles.

If toxins and associated microbes move deeper within the body, inflammatory reactions can occur that may ultimately affect the nervous system; either chronically as with ADHD, Autism, ME, or acutely with meningitis, encephalitis, poliomyelitis etc.

CHAPTER TEN

10 Herd Immunity - An emotional Weapon Based on Science Fiction

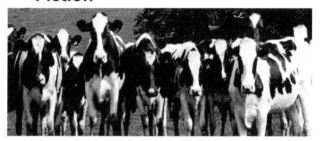

Chapter 9 Contents:

9.1 What is Herd Immunity?

9.2 Microbes Can Exist in People That Have No Disease

9.3 Vaccines Have Been Shown To Increase Disease

9.4 Vaccines Have Promoted New Strains of Microbes

9.5 Vaccines Have Never Been Shown To Eradicate Disease

10.1 **What is Herd Immunity**

Traditional View:

The orthodox view of infectious disease, used in the concept of herd immunity, implies that illnesses can only be caused by the transfer of disease microbes to an individual from someone that already has the illness.

If people are immune to the disease then they will not transfer those disease microbes to anyone else. Therefore when sufficient numbers of people are immune, the illness will die out because there are not enough carriers to give the disease microbes to others.

In such circumstances there may be a small percentage of people that are not immune and they can be protected by the immune effect of the majority, the *'herd effect'*, simply because there are insufficient numbers of people to keep the disease going and therefore virtually no one to get the disease from. So it is important that as many people as possible are vaccinated to create the 'herd effect' and protect individuals that are too sick to be vaccinated.

In addition, with sufficient vaccine uptake, illnesses can be eradicated from the world's population. It is thought that people deciding not to vaccinate are taking advantage of the herd effect for themselves, but they are also at greater risk of catching illnesses and therefore passing them on to the individuals that are too sick to be vaccinated. These sick individuals that are unable to be vaccinated are also more likely to suffer serious complications from the illnesses.

Independent View:

2. Microbes Can Exist in People That Have No Disease

The 'herd effect' from vaccinated populations only makes sense if the microbes responsible for the disease are unable to exist on vaccinated individuals. Vaccines cannot eradicate microbes from all the membranes and spaces of the human body and no vaccine producer would ever claim that or be able to prove that.

Microbes will always be present whether people are vaccinated or not. We know that many people are carriers even though they do not have the symptoms of illness.

Therefore the potential for illness always exists and the theory of vaccine herd immunity is fundamentally flawed. This is why even within highly vaccinated populations infectious illnesses still occur.

"Many outbreaks (measles) have occurred among school-aged children in schools with vaccination levels above 98%. These outbreaks have occurred in all parts of the country."

'The Morbidity and Mortality Weekly Report' (MMWR) CDC 13/01/89-38(1); 11-14

10.2 Vaccines have been shown to increase disease

Also, rather than vaccines reducing the risk of illness by the herd effect, some studies show that there is a higher incidence of the actual illness in vaccinated than in non-vaccinated groups.

In a review of a study on the BCG vaccine against Tuberculosis; not only did the results show <u>no evidence of a protective effect</u>, but slightly <u>more tuberculosis cases appeared in vaccinated</u> than in the equal sized placebo control group

Lancet Jan 12 1980

10.3 Vaccines have promoted new strains of microbes

In addition other studies show that even more serious illnesses can be associated with the vaccinated individuals than the non-vaccinated.

> *It has been reported that by vaccinating with polio vaccine subsequent illnesses are associated with new viruses e.g. echo and coxsackie viruses, which may be more severe than the poliovirus displaced by the vaccines.*

The Lancet, 1962:548-51

Therefore rather than providing a protective herd effect, vaccines could be increasing the risk of disease in the population.

10.4 Vaccines have never been shown to eradicate disease

Vaccine promoters claim that smallpox was eliminated through the herd effect of vaccination, however, we know that large proportions of the world's population were not vaccinated against smallpox.

Vaccine promoters argue that it is critical to achieve a very high vaccine uptake rate to benefit from herd immunity and to eradicate a disease. So how was it possible for the smallpox vaccine to have eradicated smallpox?

"The disappearance of smallpox from many regions despite the continued presence of large numbers of unvaccinated susceptibles was evident from the historical record (as had been noted by Farr more than a century ago)."

Paul E.M. Fine Epidemiologic Reviews
1993 John Hopkins University, Vol. 15, No. 2

Similarly why is it when we now have higher vaccine uptake rates, better distribution, better storage, refrigeration and supposedly more effective vaccines, we have been unable to eliminate any disease since the decline of smallpox?

In summary, vaccine herd immunity is a hypothetical concept that cannot be observed in the real world of disease and is completely illogical given our current understanding of how microbes live in the human body.

CHAPTER ELEVEN

11 The Polio Vaccine

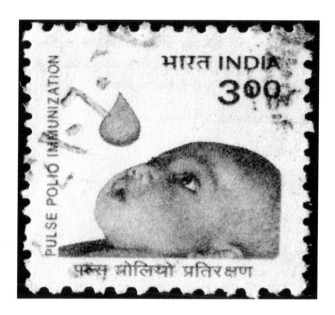

Chapter 11 Contents:

11.1 **Susceptibility to Polio**

The Polio story is a very good example of the issues surrounding microbes, infectious illness and vaccines.

Polio cases did not follow the usual trend as with other diseases such as, measles, whooping cough and diphtheria. Polio epidemics of the 1950s were occurring in the developed countries – USA and Europe. There were a number of factors that appear to have contributed to the rise in cases at that time:

1. Exposure to DDT poisoning

2. Routine tonsillectomies

3. Removal of the appendix

4. History of antibiotic use

5. High dietary intake of sugar

6. Other vaccines given can provoke polio in the recipient

Polio virus, which supposedly causes paralytic poliomyelitis, is from a family of gut enteroviruses that are actually in all of us. The disease paralytic poliomyelitis used to be called infantile paralysis or acute flaccid paralysis.

The disease is distinctly caused by neurological poisoning as determined by orthodox research in the 40s, 50s and 60s, poisoning due to the advent of insecticides DDT and DDE. It was also noted as early as the 1900s after the use of lead arsenate in the dairy industry. Note that this was not an alternative view at the time and in fact it was renowned to be NOT an infectious disease but a neurological poisoning.

As the insecticides were banned the illnesses diminished, where they continue to be used in developing countries to this day, the illness persists.

They were found to be more severe in children with compromised immune systems i.e. children with: tonsils and/or appendix removed (the tonsils and appendix are a necessary part of our lymphatic system, not an unnecessary tissue as once believed); a history of antibiotic use (antibiotics upset the important micro-organism balance within the body); exposure to lots of refined sugar (affects the blood metabolism, liver and pancreas making us more susceptible to blood toxicity problems); recent administration of other vaccines (this presents an immune shock which adds to the levels of toxins the body has to deal with).

All of which understandably pre-disposes children to invasive toxicity i.e. Illnesses such as polio that affect the brain and nervous system.

11.2 **Looking For a Microbe to Blame**

During this time however, there were other research scientists determined to find a causative microbe in the cases of acute flaccid paralysis and infantile paralysis, so that ultimately they could produce a vaccine.

From the poisoned tissue of victims, amongst all manner of debris and toxins, they found polio viruses which have since been promoted as the cause of paralytic illnesses, later to be renamed paralytic poliomyelitis. Though never proven to be the cause of paralytic illness, nevertheless the polio vaccine was produced in its various forms to counter the illness.

The vaccine has never been responsible for diminishing cases of neurological poisoning which is the true nature of what we now call polio. The illness was hijacked by vaccine producers and its efficacy has never been demonstrated, the virus has never been demonstrated as causing the tissue to become diseased in the natural illness, no infectosomes (viruses entering the cell) have ever been found or photographed using electron microscopes.

There have been two types of polio vaccine, oral and injectable and producers from both sides have accused the other of causing more polio than preventing. In fact polio vaccines, along with all other vaccines, add to the immune load predisposing individuals to more invasive illness i.e. illnesses affecting brain and nerve function.

11.3 **Polio and Swimming Pools**

The question of swimming pools often arises, is it possible to contract polio from a pool? In theory you can get any gut microbe from a pool, but you would have to ingest the excrement of another individual to be affected.

In such instances the microbe would be the last of your worries, there are plenty of toxins in human excrement that would create a problem, and your reaction would not be paralytic poliomyelitis. In fact polio has never been contracted from any pool in the UK, and if microbes were to survive in a pool, then this would be evidence of a poorly maintained pool and many other reactions would occur before anything resembling paralytic poliomyelitis.

It has been reported that individuals in a household have contracted polio from a child recently taking an oral polio vaccine through contamination of the child's excrement. However this highlights the toxic nature of the oral vaccine, the symptoms of the individual are polio-like but do not lead to long term neurological consequences, this could only happen if the individual is immune-compromised and has their symptoms acutely suppressed. In any event any household that regularly ingests their child's excrement has a hygiene issue (toxins) and will obviously be susceptible to illness.

Polio virus is associated with a whole host of symptoms from very few, to digestive complaints, to spasm, to paralysis, to brain disorder, to death, the virus is exactly the same in all cases the difference is the susceptibility of the patient. You can't catch paralytic poliomyelitis you develop the susceptibility to it from severe poisoning and immune suppression over a period of time, even if you can transfer viruses from person to person you can only develop the illness that reflects your own susceptibility.

CHAPTER TWELVE

12 The Tetanus Vaccine

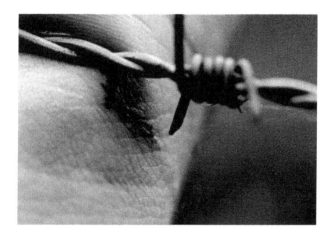

12.1 Tetanus the Illness

12.2 Preventing Tetanus

12.3 The Immune Response to Tetanus

12.4 What does the Tetanus Vaccine do?

12.1 Tetanus – The Illness

Tetanus seems to create a separate issue; the illness is caused by the activity of microbes in a cut and therefore, unlike other illnesses, appears to be more closely related to the procedure of vaccination. The tetanus bacteria themselves are widespread and can be found in soil, dust, manure, rust and even in the digestive tract of some people.

However the issues are the same, firstly the symptoms of tetanus; paralysis and rigidity, are due to poisoning of the nervous system, often the first signs are in the jaw, hence the term lock-jaw. This nerve poisoning is in fact the end result of a disease process that can be avoided once we are clear about the causes.

If a wound contains enough material for bacteria to live on, is covered, with no access to air, then the bacteria will grow without oxygen (anaerobically) this could give rise to the bacterial toxin that could lead to blood poisoning.

12.2 Preventing Tetanus

Therefore shallow cuts and grazes do not pose such a problem and in deeper injuries the first preventative would be wound cleaning; this does not require topical antibacterial treatments as the presence of bacteria are not a problem, so long as the debris that they live off are removed. Thus wound cleansing has been recommended in Accident and Emergency departments utilizing tap water only. A drugs and therapeutics bulletin, 25 November 1991, states that antibacterial applications actually slow wound healing making the situation worse, therefore tap water is recommended even in these hospital departments.

12.3 The immune response to tetanus

But, if for example, a wound did contain debris, bacteria and no oxygen, then the patient would experience a local blood poisoning, in which case the site would become inflamed. I.e. there would be an intense inflammatory reaction to the wound with the associated redness, swelling and pain.

Almost all patients in developed countries would react successfully to such a wound, unless severely immune compromised for example, patients on chemotherapy (immune suppressive drugs) for cancer.

In fact tetanus is virtually unheard of in developed countries, vaccines however cannot be used as the reason for this as it is estimated that at least 40% of these populations do not have up-to-date vaccines of tetanus. In the building industry where this figure may be higher and the nature of these wounds is a common everyday occurrence, there is no tetanus. Clearly natural immunity plays a significant role in preventing this illness.

But if a deep wound was not cleaned, and there were sufficient bacteria and debris in the wound, and the wound was covered allowing in no oxygen and the patient was unable to exhibit a successful inflammatory response, then a blood poisoning would develop with concomitant symptoms.

But this can also be treated, the wound can be surgically cleaned, the bacteria are sensitive to penicillin and there are many alternative treatments for this as well as effective nutritional advice that will help alleviate the problem.

If however this blood poisoning was not dealt with successfully i.e. if in fact the symptoms were suppressed i.e. the inflammation was suppressed then the poison could become invasive and ultimately affect the nervous system.

A passive vaccine i.e. tetanus antibodies can be given to help 'marker' the tetanus toxins that could help your response in an acute instance of toxin overload. But the body will still have the job of eliminating this poison from the system, there is also no guarantee that the body will not react to these foreign antibodies increasing the immune load as opposed to helping.

In such an instance of an acute problem, when you already have an injury, this passive vaccine of antibodies is used, but is a different type of vaccine used than in for example the DPT where you are given a weakened form of the toxin so that you produce your own antibodies whilst you are not ill.

So there are in fact a whole host of reactions and systems that come into play so that toxins from injuries do not become invasive and affect the nerves, this is actually what the body is designed to do. The risk of this illness is more or less negligible in the developed world, unless the individual is already severely immune compromised with poor wound hygiene and poor disease management.

12.4   What does the tetanus vaccine do?

But the question still remains; could the vaccine help? Once again we are back to all of the issues raised previously. The vaccine does not promote a full immune response and the associated symptoms i.e. the immune 'responses' to the vaccines are usually suppressed. Vaccines poison the internal systems directly, going straight into the blood and remain there adding to the internal toxicity (the very cause of illnesses like tetanus and polio), increasing the immune burden and the possibility of creating long-term effects.

It has been demonstrated that the immune response to tetanus results in a low T-cell response (high T-cell suppressors compared to T-cell helpers) and a high B-cell antibody response which may persist. Such a response is similar to the immune compromised response of patients with AIDS, and therefore research on the tetanus vaccine may implicate vaccines as a cause of some immune compromised reactions rather than enhanced immune responses.

As such the tetanus issue runs parallel to all invasive consequences of any so-called infectious disease.

Any illness can become invasive, whether they are diseases of the lungs, skin, and digestive tract or from injuries etc. Whatever the point of entry, the issue is the same, if the invading toxins are not dealt with, then the consequences may eventually affect the nervous system and could lead to the death of the patient.

This makes tetanus no different from any other infectious illness; measles, mumps, flu, polio, etc. and therefore the vaccine just as potentially hazardous because the vaccines tend to add to the internal immune burden.

CHAPTER THIRTEEN

13 Travel Vaccines

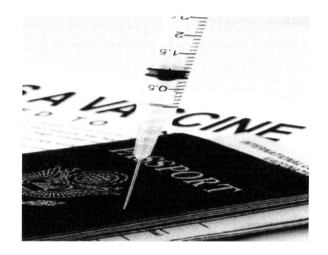

13.1 Travel and Disease Conditions

13.2 Can there be Disease without Disease Conditions?

13.1 **Travel and Disease Conditions**

So how does this compare to the issue of travel, where we supposedly have not seen these foreign germs (microbes) before? Remember the immune system does not work according to whether you have seen the germ before, like learning to cross a different road in a different country you don't have to teach your child the process all over again. So the issue is not the germ, remember the germs are the result of disease, the causes of disease are the stresses of our environment and in foreign travel there are plenty of new conditions that we may have never seen before or may not be well adapted to when we travel.

These conditions may be difficult to adapt to given the speed of travel and the short duration of most holidays abroad which can therefore lead to symptoms, from the conditions of; toxicity, different foods, different weather, different stresses, sometimes more stress, often less stress on holiday. For example adrenalin is a natural immune suppressor; work, financial/family anxieties, tea, coffee, cigarettes are just a few examples of the conditions to which we respond with adrenalin. There are many adrenalin junkies that are therefore constantly suppressing their immune activity, which is what adrenalin does (it is a natural immune suppressor). Go on holiday then the adrenalin diminishes and the immune system starts to repair and eliminate, we then experience symptoms of illness and we see that many people only fall ill as soon as they start their holiday.

Jet lag, partying, late nights, alcohol, drugs and dehydration, we see symptoms and we suppress with anti-inflammatories, anti-diarrhoeal drugs, pain killers, and headache tablets. If we notice what happens to us, we understand why we respond the way we do, suppression of responses will lead to invasive toxins, we then find a bug and we say 'ah ha... that was the cause of my illness'.

The microbe was not the cause and a vaccine could not have prevented it. In fact travel vaccines will poison the blood and will predispose you to more illness which is why vaccinated individuals get sicker and why there are no placebo-controlled trials to show the true effects of vaccines.

13.2 Can there be Disease without Disease Conditions?

But what about dangerous viruses that get you even if you are healthy, for example the Ebola virus? Yes, another fantasy, an illness so devastating, caused by a virus capable of killing anyone in its path, at least that's what the public have been led to believe and yet we have no treatment or vaccine for, which raises the question, why hasn't it killed everyone in its path?

The source of the virus is unknown; therefore quarantine would only be possible once the patient had symptoms, why is the disease not spreading from whence it came? A quote from the Centre for Disease Control (special pathogens branch) sheds a different light;

> '... *Researchers do not understand why some people are able to recover and some do not'.*

Once again some people are susceptible and most are not, in fact the illness is prevalent in hospital settings and without further research I do not know what the pre-disposing factors are, but this is an illness like all other illnesses, you cannot travel to an area of virus but an area with certain conditions, you react to the conditions, if reactions are successful no illness is possible, regardless of the presence of virus. If responses are not successful, then increasing health is required, suppression may add to the problem and you need to understand the conditions in order to lighten the load on the patient.

Microbes are always present and they change according to the conditions you are subjected to. Severe septicaemia and bacterial proliferation as a result of toxicity may require antibiotics but the illness needs to be addressed or more of the same will result, vaccines address none of the issues relating to disease susceptibility.

CHAPTER FOURTEEN

14 Is this a Minority View Held by Alternative Practitioners Only?

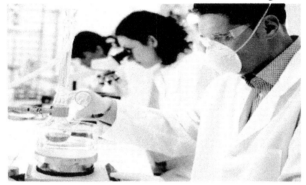

14.1 Top Scientists Questioning Vaccines

14.2 Vaccines and Autism

14.3 Cervical Cancer Vaccine, Causing Deaths

14.4 Vaccine Additives and Brain Damage

14.5 Top Scientists Refuse Vaccines for their own Family

14.6 Head Government Vaccine Assessor, Speaks Out against Vaccine Damage Denials

14.7   Head   Government   Vaccine   Regulator   says "Vaccines Don't Work"

14.1   Top Scientists Questioning Vaccines

It would appear that those questioning the safety and effectiveness of vaccines are in the minority, certainly more people vaccinate than do not and the dominant medical opinion supports the use of vaccines.

However most people don't realise that many prominent scientists, vaccine researchers and government officials oppose the official guidelines on vaccines and have found evidence of vaccine ineffectiveness and dangers that the public are not being told.

14.2   Vaccines and Autism

Dr Bernadine Healy, former head of the National Institutes of Health. Member of the IOM (Institute of Medicine) in her interview 05/12/08 on CBS News:

> Dr Healy at first considered the vaccine-autism link to be "silly." But, she said, "the more you delve into it, if you look at the basic science, if you look at the research that has been done in animals, if you look at some of the individual cases, and if you look at the evidence that

there is no link, what I come away with is, the question has not been answered."

..."but a report from 2004 basically said, 'Do not pursue susceptibility groups. Don't look for those children who may be vulnerable.' I really take issue with that conclusion."

The reason why officials didn't want to look for those groups? "Because they were afraid that, if they found them, however big or small they were, that would scare the public away," Dr Healy explained.

14.3 Cervical Cancer Vaccine, Causing Deaths

Dr Diane Harper, a lead developer of the controversial Gardasil vaccine believes this vaccine, which is being recommended for teens and pre-teens to combat cervical cancer, is less effective than the common Pap smear, and that it may harm more children than it helps.

"Parents and women must know that deaths occurred,"

At the University of British Columbia, researchers Chris Shaw and Lucija Tomljenovic in the Faculty of Medicine state that the cervical cancer vaccine may lead to death among susceptible members of the population.

14.4 Vaccine Additives and Brain Damage

Chris Shaw in 2006 also discovered that aluminium additives in vaccines were causing brain and nerve damage and after his discoveries stated:

> *"No-one in my lab wants to get vaccinated … we weren't out there to poke holes in vaccines but all of a sudden oh my God we've got nerve-cell death."*

14.5 Top Scientists Refuse Vaccines for their own Family

Professor Walter Spitzer of McGill University considered Canada's "dean" of epidemiology. In a 2002 testimony to U.S. Congressional committee hearing into the safety of various childhood vaccines, stated that, based on the evidence to date involving one of the vaccine combinations under scrutiny:

> *"I cannot recommend it … for my own grandchildren."*

14.6 Head Government Vaccine Assessor, Speaks Out against Vaccine Damage Denials

Peter Fletcher, former Chief Scientific Officer at the UK's Department of Health. Dr Fletcher was also the Medical Assessor to the Committee on Safety of Medicines, and thus the very person who determined for the UK government whether vaccines were safe. Dr Fletcher has several times gone public with his concerns over vaccines, and with his frustration that;

> "... no one in authority will even admit a vaccine-related problem could be happening, let alone try to investigate the causes."

14.7 Head of International Vaccine Research, Critical of Vaccine Policy

The Cochrane Collaboration was set up in 1992 by the UK National Health Service Research and Development Program to assess trials published in peer reviewed scientific journals, the head of the Vaccines Division is Tom Jefferson, he is highly critical of the lack of proper trials conducted on vaccines - writing in the British Medical Journal he states:

> "The inception of a vaccination campaign seems to preclude the assessment of a vaccine

through placebo controlled randomised trials on ethical grounds. Far from being unethical, however, such trials are desperately needed and we should invest in them without delay. A further consequence is reliance on non-randomised studies once the campaign is under way. It is debatable whether these can contribute to our understanding of the effectiveness of vaccines."

14.8 Top Government Vaccine Regulator says "Vaccines Don't Work"

Dr Shiv Chopra was employed for 35 years by the Canadian government regulatory department, 'Health Canada', with 20 years in vaccines and antibiotic regulation and states:

"Doctors know from their clinical practice that vaccines are given to all of their patients and repeatedly ... and they still see outbreaks of all of these vaccinated diseases so they should know that vaccines don't work."

There are in fact many more medical researchers, doctors, articles and references that can be added to this story, however in this book we have intentionally focussed on the principles to help you gain a more holistic perspective of health and how vaccines, although well-meaning, are based on outdated concepts of immunity and disease.

However if research and more scientific detail is what you are after, along with an in depth appraisal of how to incorporate science and holism in your understanding of immunity, illnesses and vaccines, then we recommend the book "Vaccines – This book could remove your fear of childhood illness" available from www.vaccine-side-effects.co.uk

It is also important to realise that vaccines are not perpetuated by powerful and malicious conspirators; vaccination is just one small element of orthodox medical practice applied to a very small fraction of possible illnesses.

Vaccines are pharmaceutical products and are simply the commercial application of an outmoded view of the human body and illness. A view that is rapidly changing into one that is more holistic and equally more scientific, a paradigm that is radically transforming the way many people are practicing health-care.

15 CONCLUSION

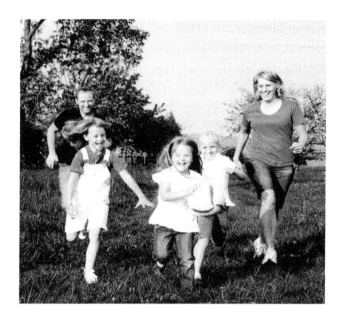

15.1 A New Health Paradigm

15.2 The Answers are in Plain View?

15.3 The Gentle and Effective Development of the Immune System

15.4 Similar Conditions Create Similar Illnesses

15.1 A New Health Paradigm

For many it takes a while to appreciate and incorporate the concepts in this health paradigm. Responsibility for our health and that of our children's health is ours and that cannot disappear by simply adopting somebody else's approach and accepting their word.

I also know that these issues can become easier and simple knowledge can be used to make the journey enjoyable. Like learning to walk; create a safe environment to allow the process and the process will happen, the consequences of failure can be greatly diminished and learning can be enjoyable.

Much of the new research (last 30 years) in immunology corresponds to the principles of holistic medicine. The immune system is a system that 'learns', hence the correlation with the brain and the mind, consequently there are scientists working within the new discipline of PNI psychoneuroimmunology.

As such the immune system learns through the small disturbances that we are subjected to, from the food we eat and the air we breathe. We do not need to create a crisis to learn. We now know that you can successfully react to immune challenges; bacteria, viruses, antigens etc. without ever seeing those substances before, just as a child is able to cross a road and let traffic pass that it has never seen before once the child has 'learnt' the basic principles and practice of road safety.

15.2 The Answers are in Plain View

So although vaccine promoters like to create fear and hysteria about **new** illnesses approaching, created by new viruses (*novel viruses*) that we have never seen before and **therefore** we have no immunity to ... they are in fact wrong.

You **do** have immunity to things you have never seen before, which is why their predictions of Sars, Bird Flu, Swine Flu, Ebola, Aids, etc. have never and will never materialise in the way they predict. Otherwise it would be obvious; whole swathes of the unvaccinated population would have succumbed to these illnesses and the vaccinated would be the ones that are surviving.

It doesn't take an expert scientist to see and understand that this has never happened. Most of the world's population have not been vaccinated against these viruses, these viruses (and increasingly newer mutated versions) are now in our environment, susceptible individuals have contracted illnesses associated with these viruses BUT most of us have never and will never succumb to these illnesses. It's patently obvious to all of us once we manage to lift the veil of confusion fuelled by the fear perpetuated by those with a vested interest in selling vaccines.

In fact it is interesting to note that the scientific research is showing the polar opposite to the dominant view perpetuated in the media. Dr Danuta Skowronski, a flu expert at the Canadian B.C. Centre for Disease Control noticed that people who had gotten a flu shot the previous year were MORE likely to succumb to the *novel* H1N1 strain, compared to those who had not received a flu shot the previous year.

Contrary to popular opinion, you can in fact be immune to all kinds of illnesses that you have never had before, through the natural development of the immune system. The specific antibody response only occurs in crisis, one of which has been artificially created by vaccination. Vaccines mimic crisis and then the reactions are suppressed, this is like accepting that your child needs to get run-over by a car in order to learn to cross the road, then trying to mimic that physiologically, just so that they react, then stopping them from reacting. As research scientists are now saying in immunology; crisis is neither necessary nor desirable.

15.3 The Gentle and Effective Development of the Immune System

Therefore we are advised to introduce foods gently to children and minimize toxins. If there are errors, reactions will be simple, we do not need projectile vomiting, inflammation and debilitating diarrhoea, but if the toxic load has been such that those reactions do happen, then that was necessary for that child. We will see that resolving illness is our innate ability and is individual, what is good for one person may not be good for another. The ability to react is important and disease is not something out there to fear or to pursue.

15.4 Similar Conditions Create Similar Illnesses

When disease conditions are similar to many people then there may be many people with a similar disease. Symptoms arise as they are required, remember diseases are 'reactions' not 'things', if we want to understand disease, understand disease conditions. In a geographical region the population is subjected to similar weather conditions, reactions such as the flu are very closely correlated to changes in weather. Illnesses will sporadically appear at identical times in individuals separated by mountains, rivers and cities and cannot have been transferred by the movement of microbes.

In an employment environment, stresses will appear at similar times, in a family there are similar conditions and similar susceptibilities due to common inheritance.

A child starting nursery will have many colds and green mucus reactions; we are often told that this is due to bugs being picked up in the nursery. However this does not make microbiological sense, there is no nursery that can contain bugs that are not already in the whole community. More importantly, children at nursery or a similar establishment, especially when this is a new environment, will undergo the stress of separation and a possible sense of abandonment.

From holistic case analysis we know that this is often accompanied by green mucus and clingy behaviour, for which the remedy could be homeopathic pulsatilla. Once the state is resolved the symptoms pass, yet the bugs are still there, as they have always been, and there are no more symptoms. We are able to help the constitution with minute doses of a remedy that is designed to help reactions, not suppress them and we are able to see what the child is reacting to, so that we may be able to reduce their load in order that they learn in a gentler manner. Part of their load is the trauma of separation from the parents.

However, those that promote the germ paradigm in isolation of the 'patient' create the sense that disease is out there to get us and the dangers of disease depend on the type of germ, whereas in reality the dangers of disease depend on the immune status of the individual. So the child is exposed to the 'disease' in the nursery, that is where 'it' lurks, other children have 'it', this mentality preys on fear, it creates more fear, we miss the obvious, and we do not learn the many causes for the disease. We feel forced to buy the drug to kill the bug, which resolves nothing, and in the process of taking the drug there has been no immune learning. Worse still, the medication may provoke some damage and if we are not aware of the disease conditions we cannot address them and we allow them to persist.

If one child has a snotty nose or a measles rash then that does not make it important for another child to have one, just as if one child vomits due to a food toxin we do not go searching for the same cause so we can all vomit. So for many of us, with sufficient information, the one remaining obstacle is our fear.

Therefore I advise you to find practitioners that understand disease, ask questions that reflect your present obstacle, ask until you are satisfied, find systems that do not prey on your fear, and learn to know how to interpret what your body needs.

If we learn to listen to ourselves we build trust, if we learn to make connections as to what disturbs us, we create a healthy environment and build compassion for life around us. If we ask the questions we need answers to, we develop from ourselves and we can pass this on to our children. Then the power disseminates from those that exploit our fear to those that would like to empower others - and hopefully we can all live happily (or at least healthily) ever after.

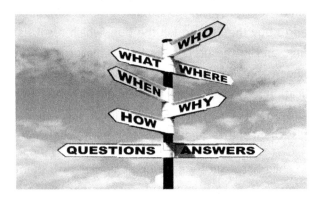

15.5 **What Next?**

You now have a number of options available if you want to deepen your understanding.

In the first instance the most obvious next step is to obtain one of the other eBooks, printed books, DVD's or online seminars in the series that is most suitable to your current needs, available from our website:

www.vacccine-side-effects.com

If you know of someone who could benefit from this information then please visit the website, go to any of the articles and simply click on email a friend.

If your issue has more to do with a specific factor that is affecting the immediate health of one of your family members but you know that the vaccine issues and concepts covered in this book will have an impact, then I would urge you to seek the services of a local holistic health practitioner that is familiar with the concepts that have been detailed within this book.

We very much welcome and value your feedback about our publications as we recognise that they can always be improved. We are committed to updating and enhancing them so that we can provide more value to the vast community of people that desperately want to find new ways to improve the health of their families. Please visit our website at **www.vaccine-side-effects.com** and tell us how we can help you further.

Yours in good health

All the team at Vaccine Side Effects

BIBLIOGRAPHY

British Medical Journal (June 7 1997; Vol. 314; 1692) [Paracetamol for fever is unnecessary].

Drugs & Therapeutics Bulletin (25 Nov 1991; Vol. 29 No.24) [Topical antibiotics for wounds do not work].

Eibl et al - New England Journal of Medicine (1984; Vol. 310(3): 198-199) [Drop in T- helper cell in response to tetanus vaccine].

Fine, Paul E.M. - Epidemiologic Reviews, John Hopkins University (1993; Vol. 15, No. 2) [The disappearance of smallpox in unvaccinated populations].

HMSO - *Immunisation against infectious disease* (1990/1996 editions). – [Comparative graphs of infectious illnesses]

Hume, E. D. - *Béchamp or Pasteur? A Lost Chapter in the History of Biology*

Mckeown, Thomas - *The Role of Medicine* [Mortality rates from infectious disease from 1850s].

Pabst, Henry – *'Kinetics of immunological responses after primary MMR vaccine'.* Vaccine (Vol. 15, issue 1, pages 10-14) [Persistent membrane leaking after vaccination].

Ronne, T - The Lancet (Jan 5 1985; 1-5) [Suppression of Measles Rash and the link with chronic disease]

Shaheen, S.O. - The Lancet (29 June 1996; Vol. 347: 9018: 1792 – 1796) [Children with a history of natural illnesses less likely to have allergies].

The Lancet (Jan 12 1980; 73-74) *Bad News from India* [Review of BCG vaccine against tuberculosis].

Thompson, William Irwin – *'Gaia 2 - Emergence: The New Science of Becoming'* 31 Oct 1991

INDEX